# Pressing RESET for Vibrant Grandparents

**original strength**

# Original strength

*Pressing RESET for Vibrant Grandparents*

Published by OS Press - Fuquay-Varina, NC


Contributor: Rob Brinkley Jr, Original Strength Certified PRO - ACE Certified Personal Trainer - ACE Group Fitness Instructor - NASM Performance Enhancement Specialist


ISBN: 978-1-963675-04-7 (paperback)

Grandparents are a gift to children.

Give yourself the gift of rediscovering the strength you had as a child by learning how to Press RESET.

Pressing RESET will allow you to express and live life to your fullest!

Imagine chasing after your grandkids in the park, feeling as agile and energetic as they are.

Imagine getting down on the floor and joining them in their games, moving freely and joyfully while still able to get up when done.

**Your grandkids are amazing!**

They jump, crash, tumble, and jump back up.
They are constantly exploring movement.
They are the opposite of fragile.

Some say, "As we age, we lose many physical abilities."

*We accept it.*
Things aren't as they used to be.

*But do you have to accept this?*

*What if you could once again tap into the wellspring of your youth?*

Think of your grandkid(s).

*How did they gain their tremendous ability to be so resilient?*

They practice and "live" in their original design!

Great news!

The child within you is still there. Your original design has not gone anywhere, it is still there, waiting for you to press the RESET button.

Think of your design as your operating system.

Your smartphone has an operating system.
If you don't reset/restart it every so often:

- Cache & cookies build-up
- Apps may be running in the background
- Its speed slows down
- Performance declines
- Commands can have a delayed response
- It can freeze up
- It can crash
- It gets glitchy

Basically, it doesn't run as it was intended to.

When you ask for advice, what question does support ask?

"Did you reset/restart it?"

Your body's operating system gets a little glitchy, too!

Pressing RESET helps you move, feel, play, and live as you were designed to!

What would you do if you had the energy and resilience of your grandkids?

Are you ready to rediscover your original design and live life better and stronger?

# Pressing
# RESET

# Original Strength's Pressing RESET Program

Pressing RESET consists of five developmental movement patterns:

1. **Belly Breathing**
2. **Head control**
3. **Rolling**
4. **Rocking**
5. **Cross-crawl movements**

(We call them The Big Five RESETS)

These developmental movement patterns restore (RESET) your central nervous system, stimulate your vestibular system, and enhance the communication between and functionality of your Nervous, Vestibular, and Muscular systems.

## Why is this important?

If your nervous or vestibular system isn't functioning optimally, your body will slow down your movement patterns. **Your brain's primary goal is to protect you,** so it will limit what it doesn't think you can do.

If your brain senses an issue, one that you may not even be aware of, this protective mechanism prevents you from functioning per your design.

The movements on the following pages are simply suggestions.

You can pick the version from each category that you like best, or you could practice multiple options from each category.

I encourage you to practice at least one movement from each category.

Play within your pain-free range of motion. In other words, do not move into pain. Pain is different from uncomfortable, you may have to push your comfort zone, but if something truly hurts, then stop. We can try something else.

Your body starts where you are.

Stay curious.

Explore your movements.

**Special Note**: Movement and Exercise have risks associated with them. Research shows that they can lead to being stronger, healthier, and happier. However, they can also lead to injuries or even death. It happens. You should also know that doing nothing also has risks associated with it. Research shows that being sedentary can lead to sickness, weakness, frailty, depression, and anxiety. It can also make you more injury-prone and hasten your destination towards death. It happens.

Before beginning any exercise program, consult your trusted family physician. You should also consult your trusted family physician before adopting any sedentary lifestyle.

"Every man dies, but not every man really lives."
- William Wallace, Braveheart

**Think back to when your grandchild was a baby and how they developed.**

# Pressing
# RESET

# Breathing (with your belly)

Remember watching your sleeping grandkids? Their bellies naturally rise and fall. Children breathe through their diaphragm (belly).

Unfortunately, many adults have developed the habit of doing more chest than belly breathing.

> **Helps you get more oxygen, calms your nervous system, and builds your "core".**

You can breathe from your chest/neck, but this is your emergency "fight or flight" breathing pattern. These breaths are typically short and shallow, sending signals of unnecessary stress throughout your body.

Alternatively, belly breathing helps you get more oxygen into your lungs, calms your nervous system, and builds your "core" strength.

# Breathing (through your nose)

Children also breathe through their noses. Do you remember how upset they'd get when their noses were clogged?

Did you ever think, "Just breathe through your mouth, like me!"

There are a lot of great things that happen when you breathe through your nose.

I'll try to keep my fitness geekiness under control and just say that your body is designed to breathe through your nose.

Imagine if you saw your grandkid as a baby, breathing shallow chest breaths through their open mouth! You'd be concerned!

But this is how a lot of adults breathe every day.

# Try this: Seated Belly Breathing

BELLY BREATHING THROUGH THE NOSE

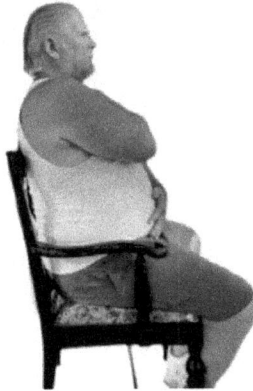

## Seated

- Place one hand on your chest.
- Place the other hand on your belly.
- Put your tongue behind your teeth.
- Inhale through your nose, filling and expanding your belly.

*Your aim is for the hand on your belly to move as you breathe.*

Set a timer for 5 minutes.

Get comfortable and start practicing.

**(or) Lying on the floor (or your bed)**

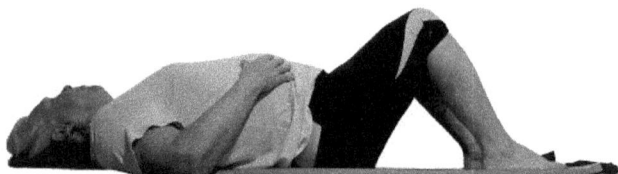

- Place your hands on your belly.
- Put your tongue behind your teeth.
- Inhale through your nose, filling and expanding your belly.

Set a timer for 5 minutes.

Get comfortable and start practicing.

# RESET #2

## Head Control

Your grandkid's heads are/were enormous in proportion to their bodies as babies!

Their heads are/were about 30% of their entire body weight.

Could you imagine if your head was still 30% of your body weight? It used to be.

Learning to move that big lunkhead around is an impressive feat of strength.

> **Movement is critical for a healthy vestibular system.**

Beyond being a feat of strength, head control stimulates and strengthens the vestibular system and helps mobilize the spine.

Your vestibular system is responsible for your balance. Every muscle in your body is connected to your vestibular system.

Movement is critical for a healthy vestibular system. The more you activate it, the more efficiently your brain communicates with all your muscles.

If practicing head movements makes you feel dizzy, stop. Instead, practice deep belly breathing until you no longer feel dizzy. Then, try again.

Start where you are and do what you can.

# Try this: Head Control (Head Nods)

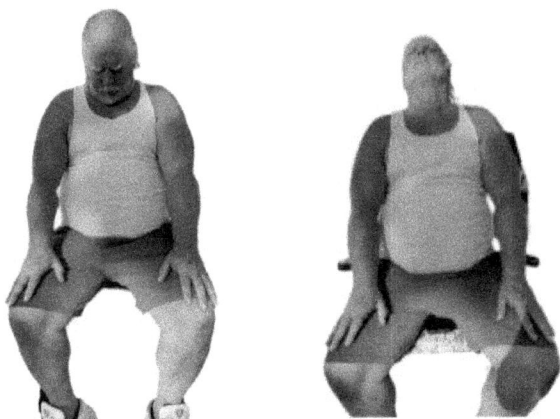

**Seated**

- Keep your mouth closed.
- Place your tongue behind your teeth.
- Breathe through your nose down into your belly.
- Move only within your pain-free range of motion.
- Lead with your eyes - look at your feet.
- Lead with your eyes - try to look above your head.

Set a timer for 1 minute and start practicing.

**(or) Lying on the floor (or your bed)**

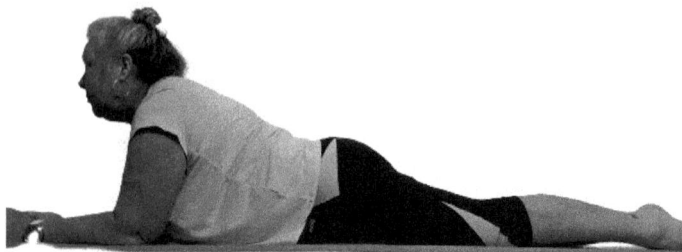

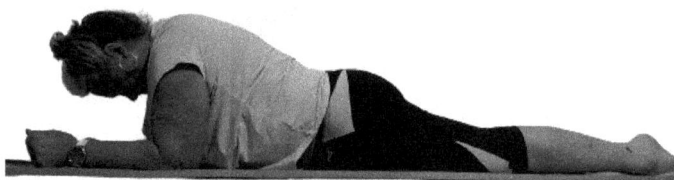

- Keep your mouth closed.
- Place your tongue behind your teeth.
- Breathe through your nose down into your belly.
- Move only within your pain-free range of motion.
- Lead with your eyes - look at towards your belly button.
- Lead with your eyes - try to look above your head.

Set a timer for 1 minute and start practicing.

# Try this: Head Control (Rotations)

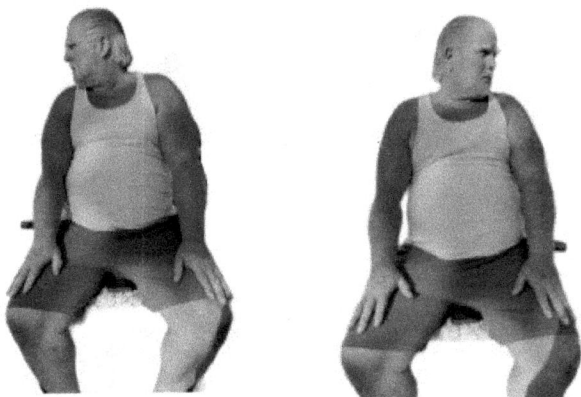

**Seated**

- Keep your mouth closed.
- Place your tongue behind your teeth.
- Breathe through your nose down into your belly.
- Move only within your pain-free range of motion.
- Lead with your eyes - look to your left, and rotate your head and neck left.
- Lead with your eyes - look to your right, rotate your head and neck right.

Set a timer for 1 minute and start practicing.

**(or) Lying on the floor (or your bed)**

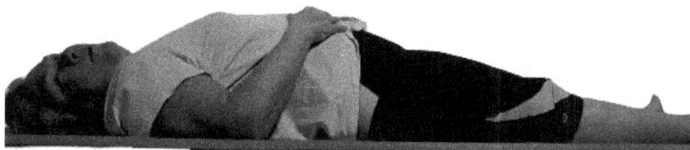

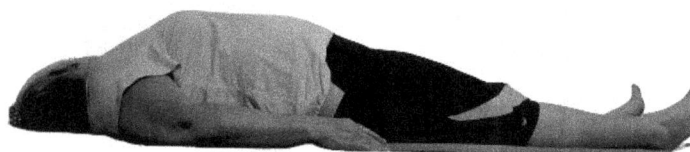

- Keep your mouth closed.
- Place your tongue behind your teeth.
- Breathe through your nose down into your belly.
- Move only within your pain-free range of motion.
- Lead with your eyes - look to your left, and rotate your head and neck left.
- Lead with your eyes - look to your right, rotate your head and neck right.

Set a timer for 1 minute and start practicing.

# RESET #3

# Rolling

Before your grandkids could crawl, if they wanted something, they rolled to it. You did this, too!

Rolling is more than just a cool way for babies and the pandas in Kung Fu Panda 3 to get around.

## Benefits of Rolling:

- Rolling ties together your opposite shoulder to your opposite hip.
- It nourishes and strengthens your spine.
- Stimulates your skin, fascia, and muscles.
- Activates your vestibular system.

The next few pages provide a few gentle options for getting back into rolling. Try them all, see which works best for you, and then practice.

> Nourishes and strengthens your spine.

Set a timer for 1 -2 minutes and start practicing.

*Reminder: If rolling makes you dizzy, stop. Spend some time deep belly breathing until you do not feel dizzy.*

# Try this: Egg Roll

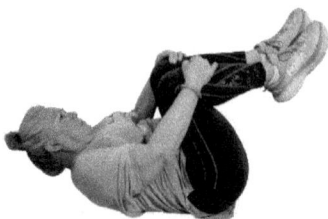

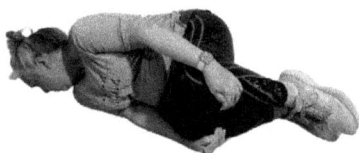

- Lie on your back.
- Hold your knees toward your chest.
- Look with your eyes, then your head, in the direction you want to go, and allow your body to roll in that same direction.
- If it feels okay, continue rotating your neck until you are looking behind yourself.
- Keep your tongue on the roof of your mouth, your mouth closed, and breathe through your nose into your belly.
- Repeat on the other side, alternating sides with each repetition.

Imagine yourself gently rolling from side to side.

*Tip: You may be able to do this in your bed; just don't roll off the bed!*

# Try this: Chair Roll

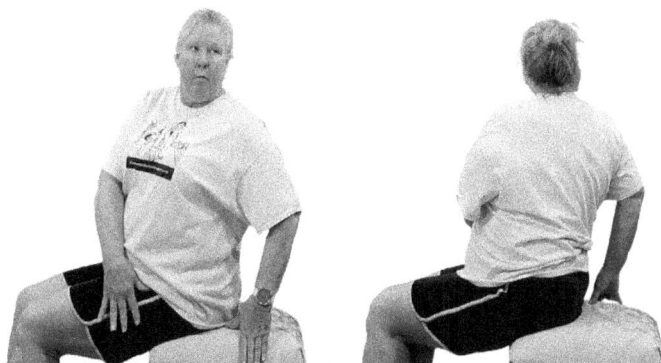

- Sit towards the front of a sturdy chair.

- Try to take a wide stance with your legs.

- Look with your eyes, then your head, in the direction you want to go and allow your body to rotate in that same direction.

- Keep your tongue on the roof of your mouth, your mouth closed, and breathe through your nose into your belly.

- Repeat on the other side, alternating sides with each repetition.

Imagine yourself gently rolling from side to side.

*Tip: You can use your hands on the chair for extra stability or to allow you to rotate a little more.*

Stay within your pain-free wheelhouse.

# Try this: Windshield wipers (rotation)

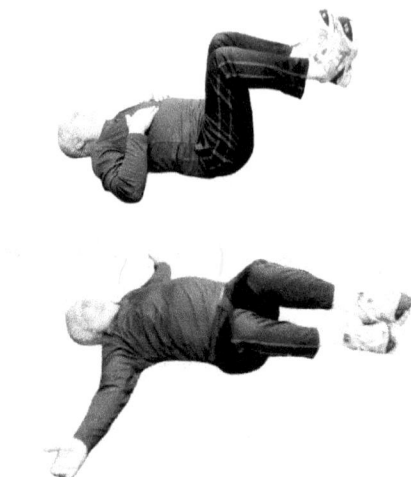

- Lie down on the floor (or your bed).
- Arms can reach out straight; keep your shoulder blades down.
- Rotate your legs from side to side.
- Keep your tongue on the roof of your mouth, your mouth closed, and breathe through your nose into your belly.
- Alternating sides with each repetition.

*Tip:* *You can pull your knees toward your chest (which may feel better on your lower back) or position them at a 90-degree angle, with your knees directly above your hips, as shown.*

Alternatively, the feet can be on the floor (think gym class sit-up position), and the sides of the legs can rotate to the floor.

# Rocking

Rocking is where your grand-kid(s) build their strength to crawl and ultimately walk.

You used to rock, too!

Great news: there is no age limit on rocking.

> Rocking gently strengthens your muscles and joints, promoting stability and coordination.

## Benefits of Rocking:

- **Activates the Vestibular System:** Rocking stimulates your vestibular system, which is crucial for balance and spatial awareness.

- **Creates Gentle Strength:** Rocking gently strengthens your muscles and joints, promoting stability and coordination.

- **Establishes Reflexive Posture:** Rocking helps establish and maintain a reflexive posture, supporting the natural curves of your spine and improving overall posture.

By incorporating rocking into your routine, you tap into the foundational movements of development and enhance your balance, strength, and posture.

# Try this: Rocking Exercise

**(FLOOR OR YOUR BED)**

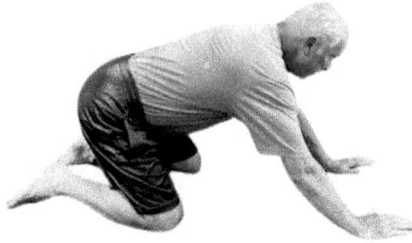

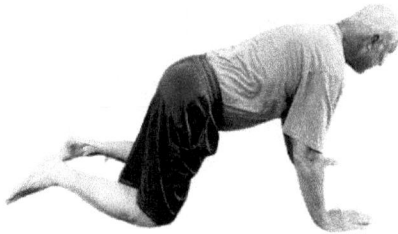

- Gently get down on your hands and knees.
- You can use padding for your knees if necessary.
- Look at the horizon with your mouth closed, breathing in through your nose and filling your belly with your breath.
- Move only within your pain-free range, reaching your hips back toward your feet.
- Then rock back to your starting position.
- Repeat the rocking motion.

Practice for 2 minutes

Pressing RESET for Vibrant Grandparents

*Additional Rocking tips:*

If your knees are tender, you can put a thick mat or couch cushion under your shins (the part of your leg below your knee), something that lifts your kneecap off the floor.

Example:

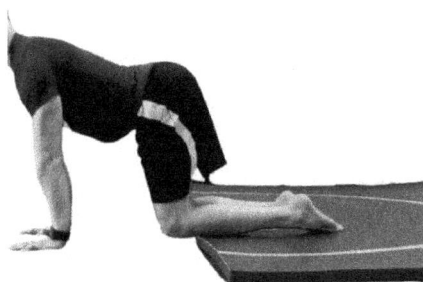

If your wrists are tender, you can use pushup handles or a couple of cans of vegetables.

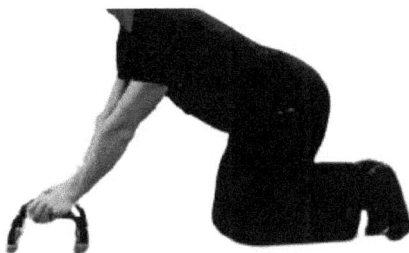

Try a few positions with your feet. First, rock on the tops of your feet (plantar flexion), as shown in the original picture.

Also, try rocking with your toes tucked under (dorsiflexion).

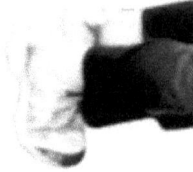

You could also explore different widths (how close your legs are to each other).

Keep your head up.

If your neck is tight, don't force it. Start where you are. Over time, you may increase your ability to lift your head incrementally.

# Cross Crawl Movements

When your grandkid(s) started crawling, they naturally paired their opposite limbs (right arm-left leg & left arm-right leg).

The crawling position offers extra benefits, such as strengthening muscles, improving posture, and providing further vestibular stimulation.

> Increases connections between the left and right hemispheres.

This patterning stimulates the brain and increases connections between the left and right hemispheres, making them smarter and stronger!

And guess what? It's not just about crawling; it works with marching, walking, running, skipping – any activity where you deliberately use all four limbs and pair opposites.

So, let's have some fun and get those brains and bodies moving together like never before!

There are no age restrictions for benefitting from cross-crawl movements. Just start where you are.

The following pages will give you multiple options to try. Be curious, play safe, and don't force anything that causes pain.

# Try this: Seated Cross Crawls

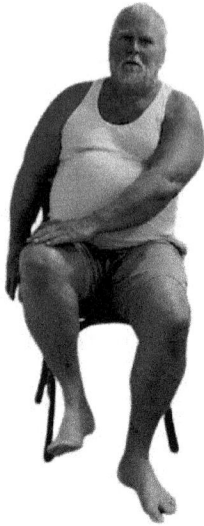

- Lift one leg.
- Touch the opposite hand to that leg (left leg - right hand).
- Switch lifted leg and touching hand.
- Continue practicing and getting comfortable with the movement. As you go, you may vary your speeds (deliberately slow, medium pace, and faster).
- Remember to look at the horizon with your mouth closed, breathe through your nose, and fill your belly with your breath.

Set a timer and practice for 2 minutes.

# Or this: Standing Cross Crawls

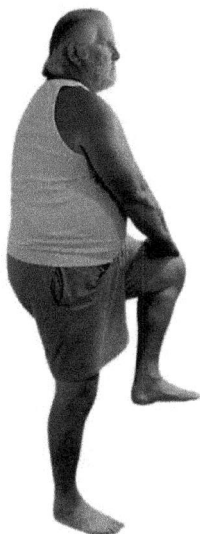

- Lift one leg.

- Touch the opposite hand to that leg (left leg - right hand).

- Switch lifted leg and touching hand.

- Continue practicing and getting comfortable with the movement. You may vary your speeds (deliberately slow, medium pace, and/or faster) as you go.

- Look at the horizon with your mouth closed, breathing through your nose and filling your belly with your breath.

Set a timer and practice for 2 minutes.

# Try this: Birddog
# (counter supported)

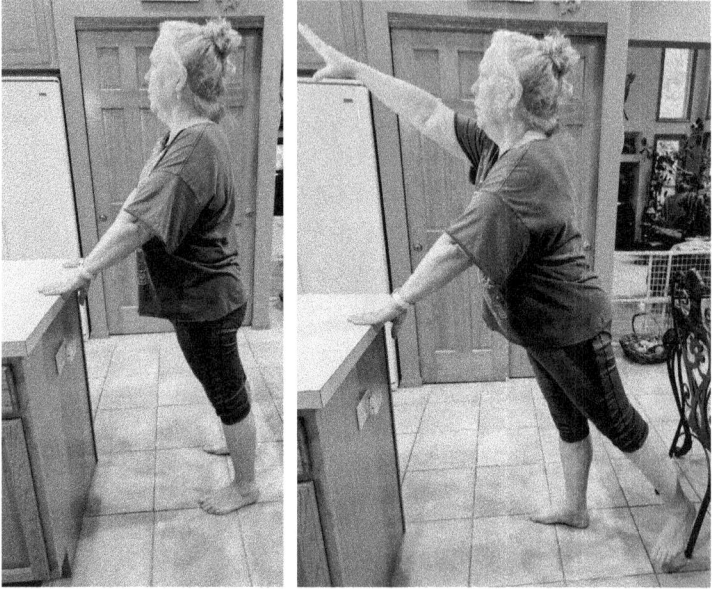

- Start with both hands supported on the counter.
- Slightly step feet back away from the counter.
- Lift one arm and the opposite leg.
- Return those limbs to your start position.
- Lift/reach with the other arm and leg.
- Look at the horizon with your mouth closed, breathing in through your nose and filling your belly with your breath.

Set a timer and practice for 2 minutes.

# Or this: Birddog (floor or bed)

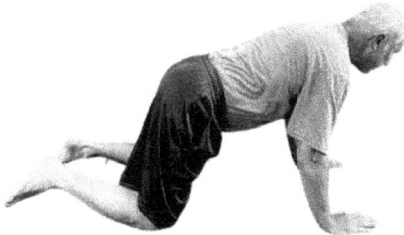

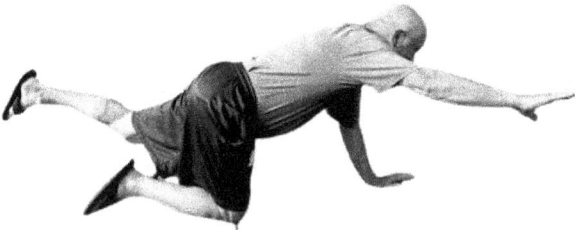

- Safely get down. Use a knee pad if needed.
- Reach one arm and the opposite leg.
- Return those limbs to your start position.
- Lift/reach with the other arm and leg.
- Look at the horizon with your mouth closed, breathing in through your nose and filling your belly with your breath.

Set a timer and practice for 2 minutes.

# Try this: Crawling

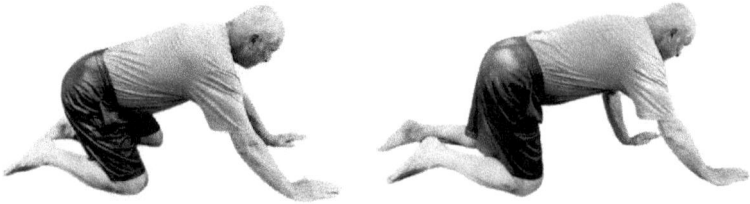

- Start in the same position as rocking.
- Crawl using the opposite arm and leg combo.
- Crawl forward using your right arm and left knee.
- Repeat left arm and right knee.
- Keep your head up. Don't force it; start where you are.
- If you have a soft surface, that could be perfect (mat, carpet, golf course-ish yard). You could also put on knee pads.
- If your wrists don't like this movement, you could use the same handles shown in the additional rocking tips.
- Breathe in your nose, with your mouth closed, tongue on the roof of your mouth behind your teeth.

Set a timer and practice for 2 minutes.

# Put it all Together:

Practicing all these developmental movement patterns will reestablish healthy communication between your muscular, nervous, and vestibular systems.

This will allow you to move better and feel better about moving!

You don't have to practice all of the included exercises. Try the ones you can. Regularly, pick at least one from each of the five developmental movement patterns (RESETS).

Keep it quick, simple, and fun.

Explore the movements. How do they feel?

How do you feel afterward?

If your grandkids are still young, recruit them to play/practice with you!

If your grandkids are older, challenge them to try it with you. Who can move more like a kid again?

Play with the movements every day.

Be creative, have fun, and always work within your pain-free wheelhouse.

# If you want a more structured practice:

Practice 1 to 3 times per day.

- ☐ Breathing (with your belly via your nose) - 5 mins
- ☐ Head control (head nods) - 1 min
- ☐ Head control (rotations) - 1 min
- ☐ Rolling - 2 mins
- ☐ Rocking - 2 mins
- ☐ Cross crawl (Marching leg tap) - 2 mins

*Tip:* *Add new (or) reinstate active hobbies that you enjoy!*

If you practice for 30 days, how do you think you will feel?

You may even notice you rekindle some old hobbies you stopped doing because you weren't feeling as great as you used to.

Others will ask you - "What's happening - how are you doing it?"

You'll have to tell them you have been Pressing RESET.

# Short Bonus:

I want to give you one bonus move to practice because I have a soft spot for Grandparents (I'll give my Grandmother credit for that).

Your bodyweight squat. Or you could think of your ability to sit and stand.

Getting up and down from a chair or the floor might seem like a small thing, but it's actually a big deal, especially as we get older.

> Being able to move easily means more freedom and independence.

Many studies show that the easier you get up and down, the better off you are.

Let's keep it simple: being able to move easily means more freedom and independence. It helps you feel less restricted and lowers your risk of falling when you stand up or sit down.

So, practice sitting down and standing up regularly – it's a small habit with big benefits for your health and independence!

# Try this: Hold the wall Squat

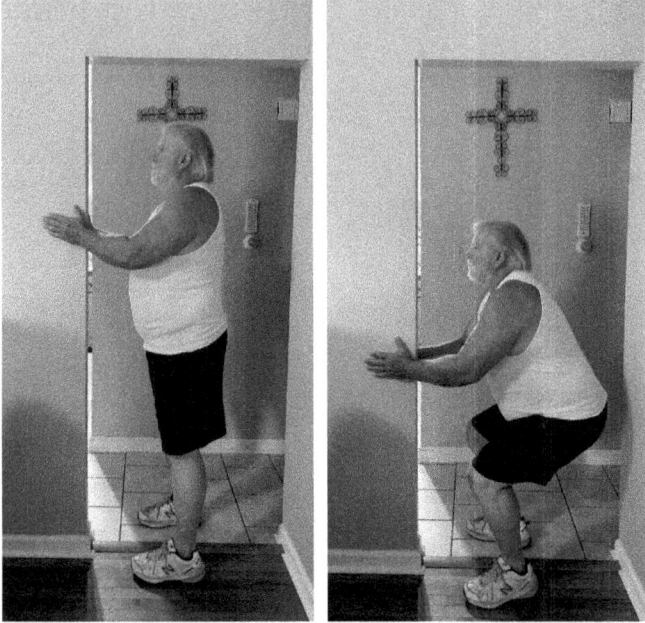

- Find a sturdy wall.

- Walk your hands down the wall as you sit your hips back, looking for a pretend chair.

- Only go down as far as you feel comfortable with your wall grip.

- Work within your pain-free range of motion.

- Your mouth is closed. You are belly breathing through your nose.

Set a timer and practice for 1-2 minutes.

# Try this: Sit to Stand

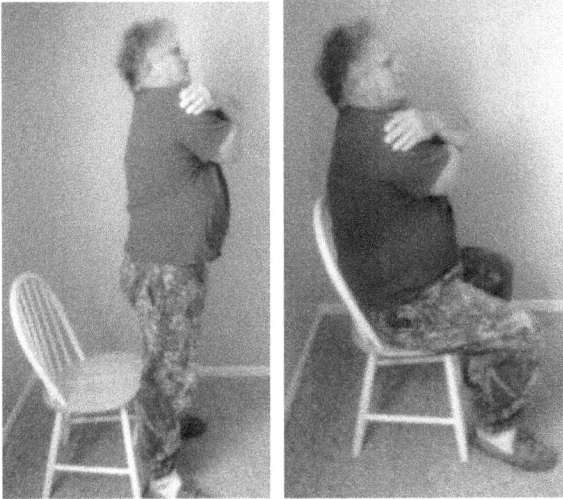

- Find a sturdy chair.
- Sit down fully under your control (don't fall into the chair).
- Work within your pain-free range of motion.
- Your mouth is closed. You are belly breathing through your nose.
- Your arms
  - » could be touching a wall for balance.
  - » could be outstretched to help with balance (in front or to your sides).
  - » could be hugging yourself to increase the challenge.

Set a timer and practice for 1 minute.

# Congratulations!

By practicing these movements, you are on your way to rediscovering your Original Strength and living life better and stronger.

Keep exploring, stay curious, and enjoy the journey!

# About Our Contributor:

Fitness has been Rob's passion for over 30 years. It all began in a Midwest basement in 1993 with lifting weights, eventually leading to competing in bodybuilding, powerlifting, and even completing five half marathons.

With 15 years of experience as a personal trainer, Rob has earned numerous certifications, reflecting his commitment to continuous learning and professional development. He currently serves as a personal trainer at the Original Strength Institute in Fuquay-Varina, North Carolina.

Rob believes in the power of movement and strength training to enhance overall well-being and quality of life. His greatest reward is helping others discover and live up to their full potential.

Connect with Rob: **robertthebrinkley@gmail.com**

# Want to learn more?

This booklet was designed to give you a brief overview of the Pressing RESET method.

We put it together because we love Grandparents. We know this booklet can help you feel better and move better. If you do nothing more than what is in this booklet, you will notice many changes in how your mind and body feel and react to various situations.

Original Strength Systems, LLC is a leading educator in nervous system restoration with a mission to bring hope and strength of movement to every body in the world. It provides quality continuing education courses and books to health & fitness and education professionals to enhance their knowledge to provide their patients, clients, athletes, and students with better outcomes.

Based on the human developmental sequence and the human body's design, OS' Pressing RESET method teaches movements that help RESET an individual's neuromuscular system, allowing them to enjoy improved physical movement and physiological function.

If you want to know more about Pressing RESET and regaining your original strength, visit https://originalstrength.net. There, you will find various books, hundreds of free video tutorials (**OS Movement**

**Snax**), and a complete listing of our courses and OS Certified Professionals near you.

If you want to improve how you feel and move, consider seeking an OS Certified Professional. They can perform an Original Strength Screen and Assessment (OSSA), a fast and straightforward method for identifying areas to unlock your potential. With the OSSA, the professional can determine the most effective starting point for your journey towards restoring your original strength through the Pressing RESET method.

Please contact the OS team with any questions you may have. *Please let us know about any changes in how you move or feel; we want to see how you are doing. Email us at Progress@OriginalStrength.net.*

**Press RESET now and live life better & stronger** because you were awesomely and wonderfully made to accomplish amazing things.

For more information:

# ⏻riginal
# **strength**

Original Strength Systems, LLC
OriginalStrength.net

PressingRESETfor@Originalstrength.net

www.ingramcontent.com/pod-product-compliance
Lightning Source LLC
Chambersburg PA
CBHW070032030426
42335CB00017B/2399